FERTILITY DIET FOR OLDER WOMEN

DR. KIMBERLY CARLOS

Copyright © 2023 by Dr. Kimberly Carlos

TABLE OF CONTENT

CHAPTER ONE

Following a Fertility Diet for Older Women with Its Benefits

Following a fertility diet for older women can potentially improve your chances of getting pregnant and having a healthy pregnancy. While it's important to remember that diet alone may not guarantee success, it can certainly contribute to your overall reproductive health. Here are some guidelines for following a fertility diet for older women with potential benefits:

1. Consult a Healthcare Professional:

Before making any significant changes to your diet or lifestyle, it's essential to consult with a healthcare provider or a fertility specialist. They can assess your specific needs, provide personalized advice, and help you address any underlying health issues.

2. Maintain a Healthy Weight:

Being either underweight or overweight can impact fertility. Aim for a healthy body mass index (BMI) by consuming a balanced diet and engaging in regular physical activity. Losing or gaining weight to reach a healthy range may improve fertility.

3. Focus on Nutrient-Rich Foods:

Include a variety of nutrient-dense foods in your diet to support overall health and fertility. These include:

- Fruits and vegetables: Rich in antioxidants, vitamins, and minerals.
- Whole grains: Choose whole wheat, brown rice, quinoa, and oats.
- Lean proteins: Incorporate sources like poultry, fish, tofu, beans, and lentils.
- Healthy fats: Include sources of monounsaturated and polyunsaturated fats, such as avocados, nuts, seeds, and olive oil.
- Dairy or dairy alternatives: Ensure you get enough calcium and vitamin D.

4. Increase Folate Intake:

Folate is essential for fetal development and can reduce the risk of neural tube defects. Foods rich in folate include leafy greens, lentils, beans, and fortified cereals.

5. Omega-3 Fatty Acids:

Omega-3 fatty acids may help regulate hormones and improve egg quality. Include sources like fatty fish (salmon, mackerel), flaxseeds, and walnuts in your diet.

6. Protein and Iron:

Iron is crucial for fertility and overall health. Consume lean protein sources, such as lean meats, poultry, and plant-based options like tofu, along with iron-rich foods like spinach and beans.

7. Limit Processed Foods and Sugar:

Minimize the intake of processed foods, sugary drinks, and added sugars. High sugar consumption can lead to insulin resistance, which may affect fertility.

8. Stay Hydrated:

Drink plenty of water to maintain optimal hydration levels. Dehydration can negatively impact cervical mucus production.

9. Manage Stress:

High stress levels can affect fertility. Practice stress-reduction techniques such as yoga, meditation, deep breathing, and regular exercise.

10. Avoid Excessive Caffeine and Alcohol:

Limit your caffeine intake and avoid excessive alcohol consumption, as they can both affect fertility negatively.

11. Consider Supplements:

In consultation with your healthcare provider, consider taking prenatal vitamins or specific supplements to address any deficiencies or unique needs.

12. Timing Matters:

Understand your menstrual cycle and track ovulation to increase your chances of conception. Fertility charting and ovulation prediction kits can be helpful.

CHAPTER TWO

14-Day Fertility Diet Meal Plan For Older Women

Creating a comprehensive 14-day fertility diet meal plan for older women involves incorporating a variety of nutrient-dense foods that support reproductive health. Keep in mind that individual dietary needs may vary, so it's essential to consult with a healthcare provider or nutritionist to tailor the plan to your specific requirements. Here's a sample meal plan:

Day 1

- **Breakfast:** Greek yogurt parfait with berries and almonds.
- **Lunch:** Grilled chicken salad with mixed greens and vinaigrette.
- **Snack:** Carrot and cucumber sticks with hummus.
- **Dinner:** Baked salmon with quinoa and steamed broccoli.

Day 2

- **Breakfast:** Spinach and mushroom omelet with whole-grain toast.
- **Lunch:** Lentil soup and a side salad.
- **Snack:** Handful of mixed nuts.
- **Dinner:** Grilled shrimp with asparagus and brown rice.

Day 3

- **Breakfast:** Oatmeal with sliced banana and walnuts.
- **Lunch:** Quinoa salad with chickpeas, cucumber, and feta cheese.
- **Snack:** Apple slices with almond butter.
- **Dinner:** Baked cod with roasted sweet potatoes and green beans.

Day 4

- **Breakfast:** Berry smoothie with spinach and flaxseeds.
- **Lunch:** Turkey and avocado wrap with whole-grain tortilla.
- **Snack:** Greek yogurt with honey.
- **Dinner:** Stir-fried tofu with broccoli and brown rice.

Day 5

- **Breakfast:** Scrambled eggs with sautéed spinach and tomatoes.
- **Lunch:** Spinach and quinoa-stuffed bell peppers.
- **Snack:** Sliced pear with cottage cheese.
- **Dinner:** Grilled chicken breast with quinoa and roasted Brussels sprouts.

Day 6

- **Breakfast:** Whole-grain pancakes with Greek yogurt and fresh berries.
- **Lunch:** Lentil and vegetable stir-fry.
- **Snack:** Raw almonds and a small piece of dark chocolate.
- **Dinner:** Baked trout with quinoa and steamed asparagus.

Day 7

- **Breakfast:** Chia seed pudding with mango and pistachios.
- **Lunch:** Spinach and feta-stuffed chicken breast with a side salad.
- **Snack:** Sliced cucumber and cherry tomatoes with

tzatziki.

- **Dinner:** Grilled shrimp skewers with wild rice and sautéed kale.

Day 8

- **Breakfast:** Whole-grain waffles with sliced peaches and a dollop of Greek yogurt.
- **Lunch:** Tuna salad with mixed greens, cherry tomatoes, and a lemon vinaigrette.
- **Snack:** Sliced bell peppers with guacamole.
- **Dinner:** Baked chicken thighs with quinoa and roasted zucchini.

Day 9

- **Breakfast:** Cottage cheese and pineapple parfait with a sprinkle of cinnamon.
- **Lunch:** Spinach and artichoke-stuffed portobello mushrooms.
- **Snack:** Fresh fruit salad.
- **Dinner:** Beef and vegetable stir-fry with brown rice.

Day 10

- **Breakfast:** Scrambled eggs with smoked salmon and whole-grain toast.
- **Lunch:** Lentil and vegetable curry with basmati rice.
- **Snack:** Baby carrots with tahini dip.
- **Dinner:** Grilled tilapia with quinoa and sautéed Swiss chard.

Day 11

- **Breakfast:** Peanut butter and banana smoothie with spinach and oats.
- **Lunch:** Quinoa and black bean salad with a lime-cilantro dressing.
- **Snack:** A handful of grapes and a small piece of cheese.
- **Dinner:** Roasted chicken breast with sweet potato and steamed broccoli.

Day 12

- **Breakfast:** Overnight oats with mixed berries and a drizzle of honey.
- **Lunch:** Chickpea and vegetable wrap with whole-grain tortilla.
- **Snack:** Sliced apple with a sprinkle of cinnamon.
- **Dinner:** Baked cod with brown rice and roasted Brussels sprouts.

Day 13

- **Breakfast:** Spinach and feta quiche with a side of fresh fruit.
- **Lunch:** Turkey and avocado salad with a balsamic vinaigrette.
- **Snack:** Greek yogurt with a handful of granola.
- **Dinner:** Grilled shrimp with wild rice and sautéed kale.

Day 14

- **Breakfast:** Whole-grain cereal with almond milk, topped with sliced strawberries and chopped nuts.
- **Lunch:** Lentil and vegetable soup with a side of whole-grain crackers.
- **Snack:** Sliced cucumber and cherry tomatoes with hummus.
- **Dinner:** Grilled chicken thighs with quinoa and roasted asparagus.

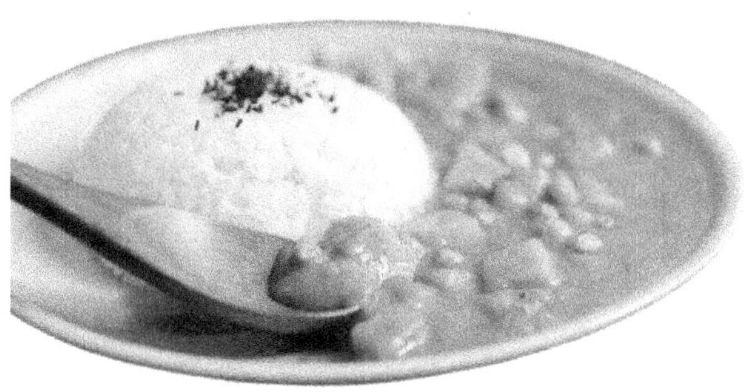

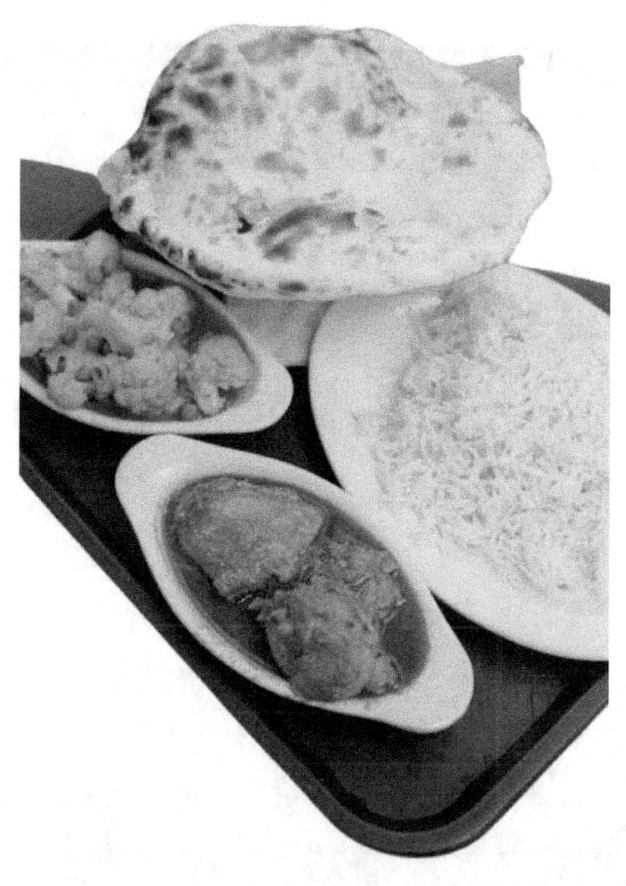

CHAPTER THREE

Fertility Diet for Older Women Breakfast Recipes

1. Berry Spinach Smoothie

This nutrient-packed smoothie is rich in antioxidants, vitamins, and iron, making it an excellent choice for women looking to boost their fertility.

Ingredients:

- 1 cup spinach leaves
- 1/2 cup mixed berries (e.g., strawberries, blueberries, raspberries)
- 1 banana
- 1 tablespoon flaxseeds
- 1 cup unsweetened almond milk
- 1/2 cup Greek yogurt (optional for added protein)

Instructions:

1. Place all the ingredients in a blender.

2. Blend until smooth and creamy.

3. Pour into a glass and enjoy!

Cooking Time: 5 minutes

2. Oatmeal with Almond Butter and Berries

This hearty oatmeal breakfast is packed with fiber, healthy fats, and antioxidants from berries, promoting fertility and overall health.

Ingredients:

- 1/2 cup rolled oats
- 1 cup water or milk of choice
- 1 tablespoon almond butter
- 1/2 cup mixed berries (e.g., blueberries, raspberries)
- 1 teaspoon honey (optional for sweetness)

Instructions:

1. In a saucepan, bring water (or milk) to a boil.

2. Stir in the rolled oats and cook over low heat, stirring occasionally, for about 5 minutes or until the oats are tender.

3. Transfer the cooked oats to a bowl.

4. Top with almond butter, mixed berries, and honey if desired.

5. Serve warm.

Cooking Time: 10 minutes

3. Greek Yogurt Parfait

A Greek yogurt parfait is a protein-rich breakfast with probiotics that can support reproductive health and gut health.

Ingredients:

- 1 cup Greek yogurt
- 1/2 cup granola (choose one with no added sugars)
- 1/2 cup mixed fresh berries
- 1 tablespoon honey or maple syrup (optional for sweetness)

Instructions:

1. In a glass or bowl, layer Greek yogurt, granola, and mixed berries.

2. Drizzle with honey or maple syrup if desired.

3. Repeat the layers.

4. Serve chilled.

Cooking Time: 5 minutes (assembly)

4. Avocado and Spinach Breakfast Wrap

This savory breakfast wrap is rich in folate, iron, and healthy fats, which can support fertility and overall health.

Ingredients:

- 1 whole-grain tortilla
- 1/2 ripe avocado, sliced
- 1 cup baby spinach leaves
- 2 eggs, scrambled
- Salt and pepper to taste

Instructions:

1. Heat a whole-grain tortilla in a dry skillet until warm.

2. In a separate skillet, scramble the eggs over medium heat.

3. Season with salt and pepper.

4. Assemble the wrap: Place sliced avocado, baby spinach, and scrambled eggs on the tortilla.

5. Roll it up and serve.

Cooking Time: 10 minutes

5. Chia Seed Pudding with Mango

Chia seeds are a great source of omega-3 fatty acids and fiber, while mango adds a touch of sweetness to this fertility-friendly breakfast.

Ingredients:

- 2 tablespoons chia seeds
- 1/2 cup unsweetened almond milk
- 1/2 ripe mango, diced
- 1 tablespoon honey (optional for sweetness)

Instructions:

1. In a bowl, combine chia seeds and almond milk.

2. Stir well, cover, and refrigerate for at least 2 hours or overnight until it thickens.

3. In the morning, layer the chia pudding with diced mango.

4. Drizzle with honey if desired.

5. Enjoy cold.

Cooking Time: 5 minutes (plus refrigeration time)

6. Spinach and Mushroom Omelet

This omelet is a protein-packed breakfast rich in folate, iron, and essential vitamins, supporting fertility and overall health.

Ingredients:

- 2 large eggs
- 1 cup fresh spinach leaves
- 1/2 cup sliced mushrooms
- 1/4 cup diced onions
- Salt and pepper to taste
- 1 teaspoon olive oil

Instructions:

1. In a skillet, heat olive oil over medium heat.

2. Add onions and mushrooms, sautéing until tender.

3. Add spinach and cook until wilted.

4. In a separate bowl, whisk eggs with salt and pepper.

5. Pour the egg mixture over the vegetables in the skillet.

6. Cook until the edges set, then fold the omelet in half.

7. Cook for another minute until the center is no longer runny.

8. Serve hot.

Cooking Time: 15 minutes

7. Peanut Butter Banana Toast

A quick and easy breakfast packed with fertility-boosting nutrients, including protein, healthy fats, and potassium.

Ingredients:

- 2 slices of whole-grain bread
- 2 tablespoons natural peanut butter
- 1 banana, sliced
- 1 teaspoon honey (optional for sweetness)

Instructions:

1. Toast the whole-grain bread slices.

2. Spread peanut butter evenly on each slice.

3. Arrange banana slices on top.

4. Drizzle with honey if desired.

5. Serve immediately.

Cooking Time: 5 minutes

8. Cottage Cheese and Pineapple Parfait

This protein-rich parfait combines cottage cheese, pineapple, and a hint of sweetness for a delightful and fertility-friendly breakfast.

Ingredients:

- 1 cup low-fat cottage cheese
- 1/2 cup diced fresh pineapple
- 1 tablespoon honey (optional for sweetness)
- 1 tablespoon chopped walnuts

Instructions:

1. In a bowl, layer cottage cheese and diced pineapple.

2. Drizzle with honey if desired.

3. Sprinkle with chopped walnuts.

4. Serve chilled.

Cooking Time: 5 minutes

9. Overnight Quinoa and Berry Breakfast Bowl

Quinoa is a complete protein and a great source of essential nutrients, while berries provide antioxidants, making this a nutrient-rich fertility breakfast.

Ingredients:

- 1/2 cup cooked quinoa, cooled
- 1/2 cup mixed berries (e.g., strawberries, blueberries, raspberries)
- 2 tablespoons Greek yogurt
- 1 teaspoon honey (optional for sweetness)

Instructions:

1. In a bowl, combine cooked and cooled quinoa with mixed berries.

2. Top with Greek yogurt and drizzle with honey if desired.

3. Refrigerate overnight.

4. Serve cold.

Cooking Time: 10 minutes (for quinoa preparation)

10. Almond Flour Pancakes with Berries

These almond flour pancakes are gluten-free and nutrient-rich, offering a delicious and fertility-friendly breakfast option.

Ingredients:

- 1 cup almond flour
- 2 eggs
- 1/4 cup unsweetened almond milk
- 1/2 teaspoon baking powder
- 1/2 teaspoon vanilla extract
- 1/2 cup mixed berries (e.g., blueberries, raspberries)
- Maple syrup (optional for drizzling)

Instructions:

1. In a bowl, whisk together almond flour, eggs, almond milk, baking powder, and vanilla extract until smooth.

2. Heat a non-stick skillet over medium heat and lightly grease it.

3. Pour small portions of the pancake batter onto the skillet.

4. Cook until bubbles form on the surface, then flip and cook

until golden brown.

5. Serve with mixed berries and a drizzle of maple syrup if desired.

Cooking Time: 15 minutes

Fertility Diet for Older Women Lunch Recipes

1. Lentil and Spinach Salad

This protein-packed salad is loaded with folate and iron, essential for fertility, and features fresh, wholesome ingredients.

Ingredients:

- 1 cup cooked green lentils
- 2 cups fresh baby spinach
- 1/2 red bell pepper, diced
- 1/4 red onion, thinly sliced
- 2 tablespoons balsamic vinaigrette dressing

Instructions:

1. In a large bowl, combine cooked lentils, baby spinach, red bell pepper, and red onion.

2. Drizzle with balsamic vinaigrette dressing.

3. Toss to combine.

4. Serve chilled.

Cooking Time: 15 minutes (for lentil preparation)

2. Quinoa and Chickpea Salad

This hearty salad is rich in plant-based protein, fiber, and fertility-boosting nutrients, making it a perfect lunch option.

Ingredients:

- 1 cup cooked quinoa
- 1 cup canned chickpeas, drained and rinsed
- 1 cucumber, diced
- 1/2 cup cherry tomatoes, halved
- 1/4 cup fresh parsley, chopped
- Juice of 1 lemon
- 2 tablespoons olive oil
- Salt and pepper to taste

Instructions:

1. In a large bowl, combine cooked quinoa, chickpeas, cucumber, cherry tomatoes, and parsley.

2. In a separate bowl, whisk together lemon juice, olive oil, salt, and pepper.

3. Pour the dressing over the salad and toss to combine.

4. Serve chilled.

Cooking Time: 15 minutes (for quinoa preparation)

3. Grilled Salmon and Asparagus

Salmon is rich in omega-3 fatty acids and vitamin D, which can support fertility and overall health when paired with asparagus in this lunch recipe.

Ingredients:

- 2 salmon fillets
- 1 bunch asparagus, trimmed
- 1 tablespoon olive oil
- 1 lemon, sliced
- Salt and pepper to taste

Instructions:

1. Preheat a grill or grill pan to medium-high heat.

2. Drizzle olive oil over the salmon fillets and asparagus.

3. Season with salt and pepper.

4. Grill the salmon for about 4-5 minutes per side or until cooked through.

5. Grill the asparagus for about 3-4 minutes, turning occasionally until tender.

6. Serve the grilled salmon and asparagus with lemon slices.

Cooking Time: 15-20 minutes

4. Spinach and Feta Stuffed Bell Peppers

These stuffed bell peppers are packed with folate, iron, and essential nutrients, making them a fertility-friendly lunch option.

Ingredients:

- 2 large bell peppers, any color
- 1 cup cooked quinoa

- 1 cup fresh spinach, chopped
- 1/2 cup crumbled feta cheese
- 1/4 cup diced tomatoes
- 1/4 cup diced red onion
- 1 teaspoon olive oil
- Salt and pepper to taste

Instructions:

1. Preheat the oven to 375°F (190°C).

2. Cut the tops off the bell peppers and remove the seeds and membranes.

3. In a large bowl, combine cooked quinoa, chopped spinach, feta cheese, diced tomatoes, diced red onion, olive oil, salt, and pepper.

4. Stuff the bell peppers with the quinoa mixture.

5. Place the stuffed peppers in a baking dish.

6. Bake for 25-30 minutes or until the peppers are tender.

7. Serve hot.

Cooking Time: 35-40 minutes

5. Tuna Salad Lettuce Wraps

These lettuce wraps are a low-carb option rich in protein, ideal for those following a fertility diet.

Ingredients:

- 2 cans tuna in water, drained
- 1/4 cup Greek yogurt
- 1/4 cup diced celery
- 1/4 cup diced red onion
- 1 tablespoon lemon juice
- Salt and pepper to taste
- Large lettuce leaves (e.g., Romaine or Iceberg)

Instructions:

1. In a bowl, combine tuna, Greek yogurt, diced celery, diced red onion, lemon juice, salt, and pepper.

2. Mix until well combined.

3. Spoon the tuna salad onto large lettuce leaves.

4. Wrap the lettuce around the filling, like a taco.

5. Serve immediately.

Cooking Time: 10 minutes

6. Sweet Potato and Chickpea Curry

This curry is full of fertility-boosting nutrients like folate and iron and is perfect for a nourishing lunch.

Ingredients:

- 1 large sweet potato, diced
- 1 can chickpeas, drained and rinsed
- 1 can diced tomatoes
- 1 onion, chopped
- 2 cloves garlic, minced
- 1 tablespoon curry powder
- 1 teaspoon turmeric
- 1 teaspoon cumin
- 1 cup vegetable broth
- 1/2 cup coconut milk (light)
- Salt and pepper to taste
- Fresh cilantro for garnish (optional)

Instructions:

1. In a large pot, heat a little oil over medium heat.

2. Add chopped onion and garlic, and sauté until fragrant.

3. Stir in curry powder, turmeric, and cumin.

4. Add diced sweet potato, chickpeas, diced tomatoes, vegetable broth, and coconut milk.

5. Season with salt and pepper.

6. Bring to a boil, then reduce heat and simmer for 20-25 minutes, or until sweet potatoes are tender.

7. Serve hot, garnished with fresh cilantro if desired.

Cooking Time: 35-40 minutes

7. Turkey and Avocado Wrap

This wrap is a protein-rich and healthy lunch option that can support fertility and overall well-being.

Ingredients:

- 1 whole-grain tortilla
- 3 ounces lean turkey breast slices
- 1/2 avocado, sliced
- 1/4 cup baby spinach leaves
- 1/4 cup shredded carrots
- Greek yogurt or hummus for spreading (optional)

- Mustard or balsamic vinaigrette for added flavor (optional)

Instructions:

1. Lay the whole-grain tortilla flat.

2. Spread a thin layer of Greek yogurt, hummus, or a drizzle of mustard or balsamic vinaigrette, if desired.

3. Layer turkey breast slices, avocado slices, baby spinach leaves, and shredded carrots on the tortilla.

4. Roll up the tortilla, securing the contents.

5. Cut in half and serve.

Cooking Time: 5 minutes

8. Spinach and Quinoa-Stuffed Bell Peppers

These stuffed bell peppers are a nutrient-rich lunch option packed with fertility-boosting ingredients like spinach and quinoa.

Ingredients:

- 2 large bell peppers, any color

- 1 cup cooked quinoa

- 1 cup fresh spinach, chopped

- 1/2 cup crumbled feta cheese

- 1/4 cup diced tomatoes

- 1/4 cup diced red onion

- 1 teaspoon olive oil

- Salt and pepper to taste

Instructions:

1. Preheat the oven to 375°F (190°C).

2. Cut the tops off the bell peppers and remove the seeds and membranes.

3. In a large bowl, combine cooked quinoa, chopped spinach, feta cheese, diced tomatoes, diced red onion, olive oil, salt, and pepper.

4. Stuff the bell peppers with the quinoa mixture.

5. Place the stuffed peppers in a baking dish.

6. Bake for 25-30 minutes or until the peppers are tender.

7. Serve hot.

Cooking Time: 35-40 minutes

9. Lentil Soup

This hearty lentil soup is rich in folate, iron, and fiber, making it a comforting and fertility-friendly lunch.

Ingredients:

- 1 cup dried green or brown lentils, rinsed
- 1 onion, chopped
- 2 carrots, diced
- 2 celery stalks, diced
- 2 cloves garlic, minced
- 6 cups vegetable broth
- 1 can diced tomatoes
- 1 teaspoon cumin
- 1 teaspoon thyme
- Salt and pepper to taste
- Fresh parsley for garnish (optional)

Instructions:

1. In a large pot, sauté chopped onion, carrots, celery, and minced garlic in a little oil until softened.

2. Add dried lentils, vegetable broth, diced tomatoes, cumin, thyme, salt, and pepper.

3. Bring to a boil, then reduce heat and simmer for 25-30 minutes, or until lentils are tender.

4. Serve hot, garnished with fresh parsley if desired.

Cooking Time: 45-50 minutes

10. Roasted Chicken and Quinoa Bowl

This balanced bowl combines protein-rich chicken, quinoa, and vegetables to create a satisfying and fertility-friendly lunch.

Ingredients:

- 4 ounces cooked chicken breast, sliced
- 1 cup cooked quinoa
- 1 cup roasted mixed vegetables (e.g., broccoli, bell peppers, zucchini)
- 2 tablespoons hummus or tzatziki sauce for drizzling (optional)
- Fresh herbs for garnish (e.g., parsley, basil)

Instructions:

1. In a bowl, layer cooked quinoa, roasted mixed vegetables, and sliced chicken breast.

2. Drizzle with hummus or tzatziki sauce if desired.

3. Garnish with fresh herbs.

4. Serve warm.

Cooking Time: 15 minutes (assuming chicken and quinoa are pre-cooked)

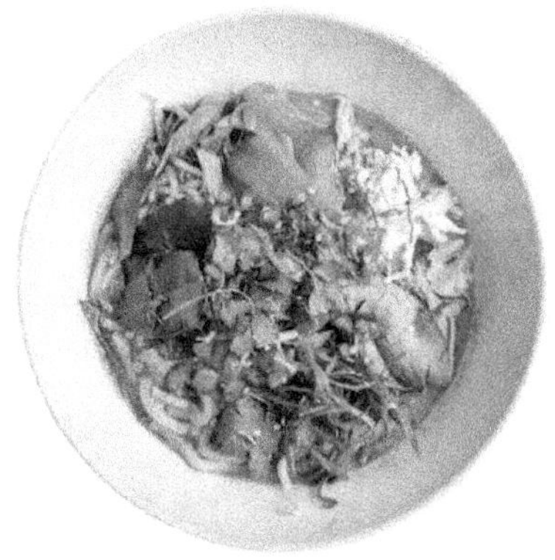

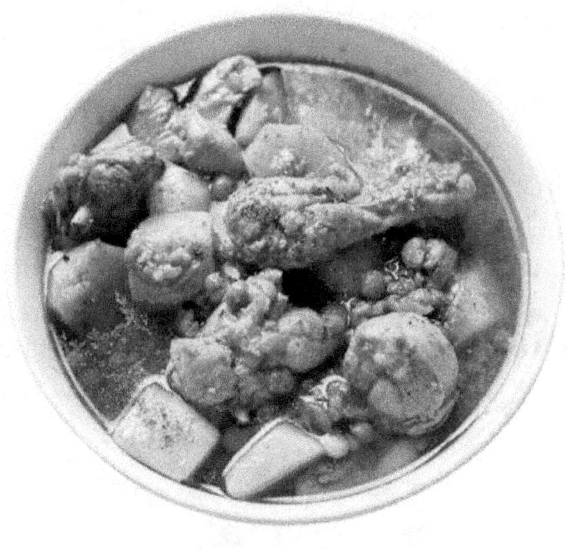

CHAPTER FOUR

Fertility Diet for Older Women Dinner Recipes

1. Baked Salmon with Quinoa and Steamed Broccoli

This dinner is rich in omega-3 fatty acids, protein, and essential nutrients, supporting fertility and overall health.

Ingredients:

- 2 salmon fillets
- 1 cup quinoa
- 2 cups water or vegetable broth
- 2 cups broccoli florets
- 1 lemon, sliced
- Olive oil
- Salt and pepper to taste

Instructions:

1. Preheat the oven to 375°F (190°C).

2. Season salmon fillets with salt, pepper, and a drizzle of olive oil.

3. Place the salmon on a baking sheet with lemon slices.

4. Bake for 15-20 minutes or until salmon flakes easily with a fork.

5. Rinse quinoa under cold water and cook according to package instructions.

6. Steam broccoli until tender.

7. Serve the baked salmon over cooked quinoa with steamed broccoli on the side.

Cooking Time: 30-35 minutes

2. Lentil and Vegetable Stir-Fry

This vegetarian stir-fry is packed with protein, fiber, and fertility-boosting nutrients from lentils and vegetables.

Ingredients:

- 1 cup cooked green or brown lentils
- 2 cups mixed stir-fry vegetables (e.g., bell peppers, snap peas, carrots)
- 2 cloves garlic, minced
- 2 tablespoons low-sodium soy sauce or tamari
- 1 tablespoon sesame oil
- 1 tablespoon rice vinegar

- 1 teaspoon honey (optional for sweetness)

- Cooked brown rice or quinoa for serving

Instructions:

1. In a wok or large skillet, heat sesame oil over medium-high heat.

2. Add minced garlic and stir-fry vegetables.

3. Cook until vegetables are tender-crisp.

4. Add cooked lentils and continue cooking for 2-3 minutes.

5. In a small bowl, whisk together soy sauce, rice vinegar, and honey (if using).

6. Pour the sauce over the stir-fry and stir to combine.

7. Serve over cooked brown rice or quinoa.

Cooking Time: 20-25 minutes (assuming lentils are pre-cooked)

3. Grilled Shrimp with Asparagus and Brown Rice

This dinner combines lean protein from shrimp with fiber-rich asparagus and whole-grain brown rice, offering a fertility-friendly meal.

Ingredients:

- 1 pound large shrimp, peeled and deveined
- 1 bunch asparagus, trimmed
- 1 cup brown rice
- 2 tablespoons olive oil
- 1 lemon, juiced and zested
- Salt and pepper to taste

Instructions:

1. Cook brown rice according to package instructions.

2. Preheat the grill to medium-high heat.

3. Toss shrimp and asparagus with olive oil, lemon juice, lemon zest, salt, and pepper.

4. Grill shrimp for 2-3 minutes per side or until pink and opaque.

5. Grill asparagus for about 5 minutes or until tender.

6. Serve grilled shrimp and asparagus over cooked brown rice.

Cooking Time: 25-30 minutes

4. Stir-Fried Tofu with Broccoli and Brown Rice

This vegetarian stir-fry is a nutrient-rich dinner option, providing protein from tofu and fiber from broccoli and brown rice.

Ingredients:

- 1 block extra-firm tofu, cubed
- 2 cups broccoli florets
- 2 cloves garlic, minced
- 2 tablespoons low-sodium soy sauce or tamari
- 1 tablespoon sesame oil
- 1 tablespoon rice vinegar
- 1 teaspoon honey (optional for sweetness)
- Cooked brown rice for serving

Instructions:

1. Press tofu to remove excess moisture, then cube it.

2. In a wok or large skillet, heat sesame oil over medium-high heat.

3. Add minced garlic and cubed tofu.

4. Stir-fry until tofu is golden brown.

5. Add broccoli florets and continue stir-frying until tender-crisp.

6. In a small bowl, whisk together soy sauce, rice vinegar, and honey (if using).

7. Pour the sauce over the stir-fry and stir to combine.

8. Serve over cooked brown rice.

Cooking Time: 25-30 minutes (assuming tofu is pressed and brown rice is pre-cooked)

5. Roasted Chicken Breast with Sweet Potato and Green Beans

This dinner features lean protein from chicken breast, vitamin A-rich sweet potatoes, and fiber-filled green beans, offering a well-rounded fertility-friendly meal.

Ingredients:

- 2 boneless, skinless chicken breasts
- 2 sweet potatoes, peeled and diced
- 2 cups green beans, trimmed
- 2 tablespoons olive oil
- 1 teaspoon dried rosemary
- Salt and pepper to taste

Instructions:

1. Preheat the oven to 375°F (190°C).

2. Place chicken breasts, diced sweet potatoes, and green beans on a baking sheet.

3. Drizzle with olive oil, sprinkle with dried rosemary, salt, and pepper.

4. Toss to coat evenly.

5. Roast in the oven for 25-30 minutes or until chicken is cooked through and vegetables are tender.

6. Serve hot.

Cooking Time: 30-35 minutes

6. Beef and Vegetable Stir-Fry with Brown Rice

This stir-fry features lean beef and a variety of colorful vegetables, providing protein, vitamins, and minerals to support fertility.

Ingredients:

- 1 pound lean beef (e.g., sirloin or flank steak), thinly sliced
- 2 cups mixed stir-fry vegetables (e.g., bell peppers, broccoli, carrots)
- 2 cloves garlic, minced
- 2 tablespoons low-sodium soy sauce or tamari
- 1 tablespoon sesame oil
- 1 tablespoon rice vinegar
- 1 teaspoon honey (optional for sweetness)
- Cooked brown rice for serving

Instructions:

1. In a wok or large skillet, heat sesame oil over medium-high heat.

2. Add minced garlic and sliced beef.

3. Stir-fry until beef is cooked to your desired doneness.

4. Add mixed vegetables and continue stir-frying until tender-crisp.

5. In a small bowl, whisk together soy sauce, rice vinegar, and honey (if using).

6. Pour the sauce over the stir-fry and stir to combine.

7. Serve over cooked brown rice.

Cooking Time: 20-25 minutes (assuming beef is thinly sliced and brown rice is pre-cooked)

7. Grilled Tilapia with Quinoa and Sautéed Swiss Chard

This dinner combines grilled tilapia, quinoa, and sautéed Swiss chard for a balanced and fertility-friendly meal.

Ingredients:

- 2 tilapia fillets
- 1 cup quinoa
- 2 cups water or vegetable broth
- 1 bunch Swiss chard, stems removed and leaves chopped
- 2 cloves garlic, minced
- 1 lemon, juiced
- Olive oil
- Salt and pepper to taste

Instructions:

1. Preheat the grill to medium-high heat.

2. Season tilapia fillets with salt, pepper, minced garlic, and a drizzle of olive oil.

3. Grill tilapia for about 3-4 minutes per side or until it flakes

easily with a fork.

4. Rinse quinoa under cold water and cook according to package instructions.

5. In a skillet, sauté Swiss chard in a little olive oil until wilted.

6. Season Swiss chard with lemon juice, salt, and pepper.

7. Serve grilled tilapia over cooked quinoa with sautéed Swiss chard on the side.

Cooking Time: 30-35 minutes

8. Tofu and Vegetable Curry with Basmati Rice

This vegetarian curry is filled with fertility-boosting ingredients like tofu and vegetables, served with aromatic basmati rice.

Ingredients:

- 1 block extra-firm tofu, cubed
- 2 cups mixed vegetables (e.g., bell peppers, peas, carrots)
- 1 onion, chopped
- 2 cloves garlic, minced
- 1 can diced tomatoes

- 1 can coconut milk (light)
- 2 tablespoons curry powder
- 1 teaspoon turmeric
- 1 cup basmati rice
- Olive oil
- Salt and pepper to taste

Instructions:

1. Cook basmati rice according to package instructions.

2. In a large skillet, heat olive oil over medium-high heat.

3. Add chopped onion and minced garlic, and sauté until fragrant.

4. Stir in curry powder and turmeric.

5. Add cubed tofu and cook until golden brown.

6. Add mixed vegetables, diced tomatoes, and coconut milk.

7. Season with salt and pepper.

8. Simmer for 10-15 minutes or until vegetables are tender.

9. Serve tofu and vegetable curry over cooked basmati rice.

Cooking Time: 30-35 minutes (assuming rice is pre-cooked)

9. Baked Cod with Brown Rice and Roasted Brussels Sprouts

This dinner combines baked cod, whole-grain brown rice, and roasted Brussels sprouts for a nutritious and fertility-friendly meal.

Ingredients:

- 2 cod fillets
- 1 cup brown rice
- 2 cups water or vegetable broth
- 1 pound Brussels sprouts, trimmed and halved
- 2 tablespoons olive oil
- Lemon wedges
- Salt and pepper to taste

Instructions:

1. Preheat the oven to 375°F (190°C).

2. Season cod fillets with salt, pepper, and a drizzle of olive oil.

3. Place cod fillets on a baking sheet and squeeze lemon juice over them.

4. Roast in the oven for 15-20 minutes or until cod is cooked through.

5. Rinse brown rice under cold water and cook according to package instructions.

6. Toss Brussels sprouts with olive oil, salt, and pepper.

7. Roast Brussels sprouts in the oven for about 20 minutes or until tender and slightly crispy.

8. Serve baked cod over cooked brown rice with roasted Brussels sprouts on the side.

Cooking Time: 35-40 minutes

10. Spinach and Feta-Stuffed Chicken Breast

This dinner features stuffed chicken breast with spinach and feta, served with a side of mixed greens, creating a protein-rich and fertility-friendly meal.

Ingredients:

- 2 boneless, skinless chicken breasts
- 2 cups fresh baby spinach
- 1/2 cup crumbled feta cheese

- 1/4 cup diced tomatoes

- 1/4 cup diced red onion

- Olive oil

- Salt and pepper to taste

- Mixed greens for serving

Instructions:

1. Preheat the oven to 375°F (190°C).

2. In a bowl, combine baby spinach, crumbled feta cheese, diced tomatoes, diced red onion, a drizzle of olive oil, salt, and pepper.

3. Cut a pocket into each chicken breast.

4. Stuff the chicken breasts with the spinach and feta mixture.

5. Season the outside of the chicken breasts with salt, pepper, and a drizzle of olive oil.

6. Place the stuffed chicken breasts on a baking sheet.

7. Bake for 25-30 minutes or until chicken is cooked through.

8. Serve stuffed chicken breast with mixed greens on the side.

Cooking Time: 35-40 minutes

Fertility Diet for Older Women Snacks Recipes

1. Greek Yogurt with Berries

This simple snack is rich in protein and antioxidants, making it an excellent choice for a fertility-boosting snack.

Ingredients:

- 1 cup Greek yogurt
- 1/2 cup mixed berries (e.g., blueberries, strawberries, raspberries)
- 1 teaspoon honey (optional for sweetness)

Instructions:

1. In a bowl, scoop Greek yogurt.

2. Top with mixed berries.

3. Drizzle with honey if desired.

4. Enjoy!

Preparation Time: 5 minutes

2. Almonds and Dried Apricots

Almonds provide healthy fats and protein, while dried apricots offer fiber and iron, making this a nutritious and quick snack option.

Ingredients:

- 1/4 cup almonds (unsalted)
- 1/4 cup dried apricots (unsweetened)

Instructions:

1. Measure out almonds and dried apricots.

2. Combine them in a small bowl.

3. Enjoy this satisfying and nutrient-rich snack.

Preparation Time: 2 minutes

3. Cottage Cheese with Pineapple

Cottage cheese is a great source of protein and calcium, while pineapple adds a touch of sweetness to this fertility-friendly snack.

Ingredients:

- 1/2 cup low-fat cottage cheese
- 1/2 cup diced fresh pineapple

Instructions:

1. Spoon cottage cheese into a bowl.

2. Top with diced fresh pineapple.

3. Mix them together or enjoy them separately for a delightful snack.

Preparation Time: 3 minutes

4. Avocado Toast with Tomato

Avocado toast is a satisfying and nutrient-rich snack, with avocado providing healthy fats and tomatoes adding vitamins and antioxidants.

Ingredients:

- 1 slice whole-grain bread
- 1/2 ripe avocado, mashed
- 1 small tomato, sliced
- Salt and pepper to taste

Instructions:

1. Toast the whole-grain bread.

2. Spread mashed avocado on the toast.

3. Top with tomato slices.

4. Season with salt and pepper.

5. Enjoy your creamy and flavorful snack.

Preparation Time: 5 minutes

5. Hummus and Vegetable Sticks

Hummus is a protein-packed dip, and paired with vegetable sticks, it makes for a crunchy and satisfying snack.

Ingredients:

- 1/4 cup hummus (store-bought or homemade)
- Assorted vegetable sticks (e.g., carrots, cucumbers, bell peppers)

Instructions:

1. Arrange vegetable sticks on a plate.

2. Serve with a side of hummus for dipping.

3. Enjoy this nutritious and crunchy snack.

Preparation Time: 5 minutes

6. Berry and Nut Parfait

This parfait combines the goodness of berries, nuts, and yogurt for a nutrient-rich snack option.

Ingredients:

-   1/2 cup mixed berries (e.g., strawberries, blueberries, raspberries)
-   1/4 cup chopped nuts (e.g., almonds, walnuts)
-   1/2 cup Greek yogurt

Instructions:

1. Layer Greek yogurt, mixed berries, and chopped nuts in a glass or bowl.

2. Repeat the layers if desired.

3. Enjoy this delightful and filling snack.

Preparation Time: 5 minutes

7. Spinach and Feta Stuffed Mushrooms

These stuffed mushrooms are rich in iron and folate, making them a fertility-boosting savory snack.

Ingredients:

- 6-8 large mushrooms, cleaned and stems removed
- 1/4 cup frozen chopped spinach, thawed and squeezed dry
- 2 tablespoons crumbled feta cheese
- 1 clove garlic, minced
- Olive oil
- Salt and pepper to taste

Instructions:

1. Preheat the oven to 350°F (175°C).

2. In a bowl, mix together chopped spinach, crumbled feta cheese, minced garlic, a drizzle of olive oil, salt, and pepper.

3. Stuff each mushroom cap with the spinach and feta mixture.

4. Place the stuffed mushrooms on a baking sheet.

5. Bake for 15-20 minutes or until mushrooms are tender.

6. Enjoy these savory and fertility-friendly stuffed mushrooms.

Preparation Time: 25-30 minutes

8. Chia Seed Pudding with Mango

Chia seeds are packed with nutrients and omega-3 fatty acids, while mango adds natural sweetness to this fertility-boosting snack.

Ingredients:

- 2 tablespoons chia seeds
- 1/2 cup unsweetened almond milk
- 1/2 ripe mango, diced
- 1 teaspoon honey (optional for sweetness)

Instructions:

1. In a bowl, combine chia seeds and almond milk.

2. Stir well, cover, and refrigerate for at least 2 hours or overnight until it thickens.

3. In the morning, layer the chia pudding with diced mango.

4. Drizzle with honey if desired.

5. Enjoy this cold and nutrient-rich snack.

Preparation Time: 5 minutes (plus refrigeration time)

9. Edamame with Sea Salt

Edamame, or young soybeans, are a protein-rich snack that also provides essential vitamins and minerals.

Ingredients:

- 1 cup edamame (frozen or fresh)
- Sea salt for sprinkling

Instructions:

1. Cook edamame according to package instructions.

2. Drain and sprinkle with sea salt.

3. Enjoy these delicious and nutrient-packed soybean pods.

Preparation Time: 5 minutes

10. Apple and Almond Butter Slices

Apples provide fiber and antioxidants, while almond butter adds healthy fats and protein to create a satisfying and fertility-friendly snack.

Ingredients:

- 1 apple, sliced
- 2 tablespoons natural almond butter

Instructions:

1. Slice the apple into thin rounds.

2. Spread almond butter on each apple slice.

3. Enjoy this sweet and savory snack.

Preparation Time: 5 minutes

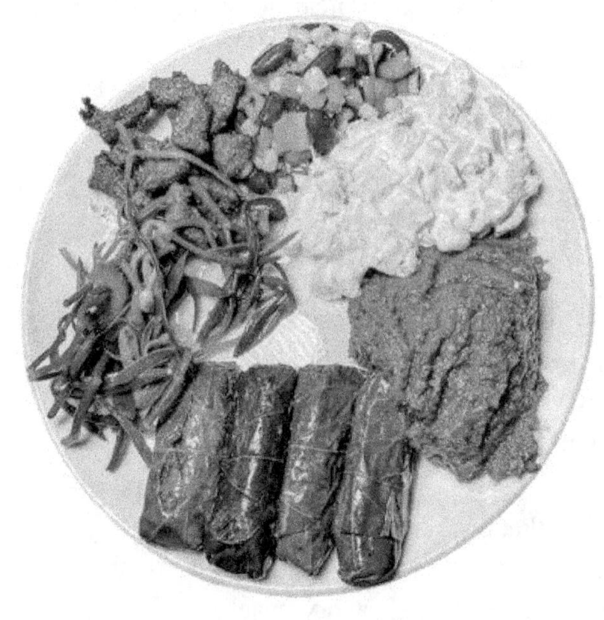

CONCLUSION

In conclusion, adopting a fertility diet can be a beneficial and empowering choice for older women seeking to optimize their reproductive health. As we age, fertility naturally declines, but nutrition plays a vital role in supporting and enhancing our chances of conception. A well-balanced fertility diet not only improves the chances of successful pregnancy but also contributes to overall health and well-being.

Key principles of a fertility diet for older women include:

1. **Nutrient-Rich Foods:** Incorporating a wide variety of nutrient-dense foods such as fruits, vegetables, whole grains, lean proteins, and healthy fats ensures that the body receives essential vitamins, minerals, and antioxidants necessary for reproductive health.

2. **Balanced Macronutrients:** Maintaining an appropriate balance of carbohydrates, proteins, and fats can help regulate hormones, blood sugar levels, and weight, all of which can impact fertility.

3. **Folate and Iron:** Foods rich in folate and iron are crucial for older women, as they support healthy egg production and prevent neural tube defects in case of pregnancy.

4. **Omega-3 Fatty Acids:** Including sources of omega-3 fatty acids like fatty fish, flaxseeds, and walnuts can reduce inflammation and improve egg quality.

5. **Adequate Hydration:** Staying well-hydrated is essential for hormone regulation and overall health.

6. **Limiting Processed Foods and Sugar:** Reducing the consumption of processed foods and added sugars can help manage weight and prevent insulin resistance, which can affect fertility.

7. **Maintaining a Healthy Weight:** Achieving and maintaining a healthy body weight is vital for fertility, as being underweight or overweight can disrupt hormonal balance.

8. **Regular Exercise:** Incorporating regular physical activity into one's routine helps maintain a healthy weight, manage stress, and promote overall well-being.

9. **Fertility Supplements:** In consultation with a healthcare provider, some older women may consider fertility supplements like folic acid, CoQ10, or vitamin D to address specific deficiencies.

10. **Stress Management:** High stress levels can negatively impact fertility. Practices such as yoga, meditation, and mindfulness can help reduce stress and promote relaxation.

It's important to recognize that individual dietary needs and fertility challenges can vary, so consulting with a healthcare provider or a fertility specialist is crucial when embarking on a fertility diet. They can provide personalized guidance and recommendations based on individual health factors and goals.

Incorporating these dietary and lifestyle changes as part of a holistic approach can contribute to increased fertility, overall health, and a higher chance of successful conception for older women. While fertility may decline with age, a well-nourished body and a positive mindset can make a significant difference in the journey towards achieving the dream of parenthood.